Created by <u>BabyDreamers.net</u>

First Printed 2023.

❤   Designed In New Zealand

Free Book Offer:

Get How to be a Super Mom For Free

A Short Read is a type of book that is designed to be read in one quick sitting.

These no fluff books are perfect for people who want an overview about a subject in a short period of time.

Table of Contents

Overcoming Common Obstacles to Getting Pregnant

Trying to conceive a child is an exciting and hopeful time for couples. However, many couples face challenges and obstacles along their journey to parenthood. Understanding these obstacles and finding solutions to overcome them is crucial for increasing the chances of getting pregnant. In this article, we will explore some common obstacles couples face when trying to conceive and discuss potential solutions.

Age is one of the most significant factors that can affect fertility. As women age, the quality and quantity of their eggs decrease, making it more difficult to conceive. It is essential for couples to understand the impact of age on fertility and explore ways to improve their chances of conception. Additionally, various health conditions can also interfere with fertility. Conditions such as Polycystic Ovary Syndrome (PCOS) and endometriosis can make it challenging to get pregnant. However, with proper management and treatment, couples can increase their chances of successful conception.

Unhealthy lifestyle habits can also have a detrimental effect on fertility. Smoking, excessive alcohol consumption, and poor nutrition can all impact reproductive health. It is important for couples to be aware of the negative effects of these habits and make necessary changes to improve their chances of getting pregnant. Furthermore, stress can play a significant role in infertility. High levels of stress can disrupt hormonal balance and interfere with the ovulation process. Implementing stress management techniques and seeking support can help couples navigate the emotional challenges of infertility.

Irregular menstrual cycles can also pose a challenge when trying to conceive. Hormonal imbalances and conditions like PCOS can cause irregular periods, making it difficult to predict ovulation. Understanding the causes of irregular periods and exploring methods to regulate the menstrual cycle can significantly improve the chances of getting pregnant. Additionally, low sperm count in men can also be a barrier to conception. Lifestyle changes, such as maintaining a healthy diet and avoiding heat exposure, can help improve sperm health and quantity.

In some cases, blocked fallopian tubes can prevent sperm from reaching the egg, resulting in infertility. Diagnostic procedures like hysterosalpingography (HSG) can identify blockages, and surgical interventions may be necessary to restore fertility. Unexplained infertility can be particularly frustrating for couples as there is no clear underlying cause. Comprehensive fertility testing and alternative therapies can help identify potential issues and improve the chances of successful conception.

For couples facing severe fertility challenges, assisted reproductive technologies (ART) such as in vitro fertilization (IVF) can offer hope. These advanced procedures can increase the chances of getting pregnant, but they also come with their own set of considerations and success rates. It is essential for couples to understand the process and options available to make informed decisions.

Infertility can take an emotional toll on individuals and couples. It is crucial to address the psychological impact and seek support from support groups and therapy. Self-care practices and stress management techniques can also help maintain emotional well-being during the fertility journey.

In conclusion, overcoming common obstacles to getting pregnant requires understanding the challenges couples face and exploring potential solutions. By addressing age-related factors, health conditions, unhealthy lifestyle habits, stress, irregular menstrual cycles, low sperm count, blocked fallopian tubes, unexplained infertility, and considering assisted reproductive technologies, couples can increase their chances of successful conception. Additionally, prioritizing emotional well-being and seeking support is essential throughout the fertility journey.

Age and Fertility

Understanding the impact of age on fertility is crucial for couples trying to conceive. As women age, their fertility naturally declines. This is because women are born with a finite number of eggs, and as they age, the quality and quantity of those eggs decrease. By the time a woman reaches her late 30s or early 40s, her chances of getting pregnant naturally are significantly reduced.

However, there are ways to improve the chances of conception, even as age becomes a factor. One option is to consider assisted reproductive technologies (ART), such as in vitro fertilization (IVF). IVF involves fertilizing eggs outside the body and then transferring the embryos into the uterus. This can be a successful option for women who are older and have a lower chance of conceiving naturally.

Another way to improve fertility is to maintain a healthy lifestyle. This includes eating a balanced diet, exercising regularly, and avoiding harmful habits such as smoking and excessive alcohol consumption. Additionally, managing stress levels and getting enough sleep can also positively impact fertility.

It's important for couples to have open and honest conversations about their fertility goals and options. Consulting with a fertility specialist can provide valuable insight and guidance on the best course of action based on individual circumstances. Remember, age is just one factor in the fertility equation, and there are still many possibilities for achieving a successful pregnancy.

Health Conditions and Infertility

When it comes to trying to conceive, various health conditions can pose challenges and affect fertility. Understanding these conditions and exploring potential treatments can help couples overcome infertility hurdles and increase their chances of successful conception.

One common health condition that can impact fertility is Polycystic Ovary Syndrome (PCOS). This hormonal disorder affects women and can interfere with regular ovulation, making it more difficult to get pregnant. However, with proper management and treatment, women with PCOS can improve their chances of conceiving. Lifestyle changes, such as maintaining a healthy weight and exercising regularly, can help regulate hormones and promote regular ovulation. Medications, such as oral contraceptives or fertility drugs, may also be prescribed to stimulate ovulation.

Another health condition to consider is endometriosis. This condition occurs when the tissue lining the uterus grows outside of the uterus, leading to inflammation and potential scarring. Endometriosis can cause fertility issues by affecting the function of the ovaries, fallopian tubes, and uterus. Treatments for endometriosis-related infertility may include surgical removal of endometrial tissue, hormone therapy to suppress the growth of endometrial tissue, or assisted reproductive technologies (ART) such as in vitro fertilization (IVF).

Male factor infertility is another aspect to consider when exploring health conditions and fertility. Issues such as low sperm count, poor sperm motility, or abnormal sperm shape can impact a couple's ability to conceive. Lifestyle changes, such as maintaining a healthy diet, exercising regularly, and avoiding heat exposure, can help improve sperm health and quantity. In some cases, medical interventions such as medication or surgery may be recommended to address specific male infertility issues.

It's important to remember that each individual's situation is unique, and seeking professional medical advice is crucial when dealing with health conditions and infertility. A fertility specialist can provide a comprehensive evaluation and recommend personalized treatment options based on the specific health condition and fertility goals of the couple.

Polycystic Ovary Syndrome (PCOS)

Polycystic Ovary Syndrome (PCOS)

Polycystic Ovary Syndrome (PCOS) is a common hormonal disorder that affects women of reproductive age. It is characterized by the presence of cysts on the ovaries, irregular menstrual cycles, and high levels of androgens, which are male hormones. PCOS can significantly interfere with pregnancy and make it challenging for women to conceive naturally.

One of the main reasons PCOS affects fertility is due to irregular ovulation or the lack of ovulation altogether. Ovulation is the process in which the ovaries release an egg, which is necessary for fertilization to occur. In women with PCOS, the hormonal imbalances disrupt the regular ovulation cycle, making it difficult for the egg to be released.

Fortunately, there are several strategies to manage PCOS and improve the chances of successful conception. Lifestyle modifications, such as maintaining a healthy weight through regular exercise and a balanced diet, can help regulate hormone levels and promote ovulation. Losing even a small amount of weight can have a significant impact on restoring regular menstrual cycles and increasing fertility.

In some cases, medication may be prescribed to stimulate ovulation. Clomiphene citrate is commonly used to induce ovulation in women with PCOS. It works by blocking the estrogen receptors in the brain, which triggers the release of follicle-stimulating hormone (FSH) and luteinizing hormone (LH), essential for ovulation. Other medications, such as metformin, may be prescribed to regulate insulin levels, as insulin resistance is often associated with PCOS.

For women with PCOS who are struggling to conceive, assisted reproductive technologies (ART) can be an option. In vitro fertilization (IVF) is a commonly used ART procedure where eggs are retrieved from the ovaries, fertilized with sperm in a laboratory, and then transferred back into the uterus. This bypasses the need for regular ovulation and increases the chances of successful pregnancy.

In conclusion, understanding how PCOS can interfere with pregnancy is crucial for women with this condition. By managing PCOS through lifestyle modifications, medication, and potentially ART, women with PCOS can increase their chances of successful conception and fulfill their dreams of starting a family.

Endometriosis

Endometriosis is a medical condition that can have a significant impact on fertility. It occurs when the tissue lining the uterus, known as the endometrium, grows outside of the uterus. This abnormal growth can cause inflammation, scarring, and the formation of adhesions in the pelvic area. These changes can interfere with the normal functioning of the reproductive organs and make it more difficult for couples to conceive.

One of the main effects of endometriosis on fertility is the disruption of the menstrual cycle. Women with endometriosis may experience irregular periods, heavy bleeding, or even the absence of menstruation. These irregularities can make it challenging to predict ovulation, which is crucial for successful conception. Additionally, the presence of endometrial tissue outside of the uterus can create a hostile environment for the fertilized egg, making it difficult for implantation to occur.

Fortunately, there are treatment options available for women with endometriosis who are trying to conceive. The approach to treatment will depend on the severity of the condition and the individual's specific circumstances. In some cases, hormonal therapies may be prescribed to suppress the growth of endometrial tissue and alleviate symptoms. These therapies can help regulate the menstrual cycle and improve the chances of conception.

In more severe cases, surgical intervention may be necessary. Laparoscopic surgery is commonly used to remove endometrial implants, adhesions, and cysts. This procedure can help restore the normal anatomy of the reproductive organs and improve fertility. In some instances, a more extensive surgery called a laparotomy may be required.

It's important for individuals with endometriosis who are trying to conceive to work closely with their healthcare provider to develop a personalized treatment plan. By addressing the effects of endometriosis on fertility and exploring the available treatment options, couples can increase their chances of successful conception and starting a family.

Male Factor Infertility

Male factor infertility refers to fertility issues that are primarily caused by problems with the male reproductive system. While it is often assumed that infertility is solely a female concern, male factors contribute to approximately 40-50% of all infertility cases. Understanding the common issues that can affect male fertility is crucial in finding potential solutions and improving the chances of conception.

There are several factors that can contribute to male infertility. One of the most common issues is a low sperm count, also known as oligospermia. This occurs when the semen contains fewer sperm than normal, making it more difficult for fertilization to occur. Other issues include poor sperm motility, which refers to the sperm's ability to swim and reach the egg, and abnormal sperm morphology, which refers to the shape and structure of the sperm.

Fortunately, there are potential solutions available for male factor infertility. In some cases, lifestyle changes can significantly improve sperm health and quantity. These changes may include adopting a healthier diet, incorporating regular exercise, and avoiding excessive heat exposure, as high temperatures can negatively impact sperm production. Additionally, certain medications or supplements may be prescribed to address specific issues, such as hormonal imbalances or low sperm count.

In more severe cases, medical interventions may be necessary. Surgical procedures, such as varicocele repair or testicular sperm extraction (TESE), can be performed to address structural abnormalities or retrieve sperm directly from the testicles. Assisted reproductive technologies (ART), such as intracytoplasmic sperm injection (ICSI), can also be used to overcome male infertility by injecting a single sperm directly into an egg during the fertilization process.

It is important for couples experiencing male factor infertility to seek professional help from a fertility specialist. A comprehensive evaluation can help identify the underlying causes of infertility and guide the selection of appropriate treatments. By addressing male infertility issues and exploring potential solutions, couples can increase their chances of successfully conceiving and starting a family.

Unhealthy Lifestyle Habits

When it comes to trying to conceive, it's important to be aware of the impact that unhealthy lifestyle habits can have on fertility. Certain habits such as smoking, excessive alcohol consumption, and poor diet can significantly decrease the chances of getting pregnant. Let's explore how these habits can affect fertility and what steps can be taken to improve the chances of conception.

Smoking and Fertility:

Smoking is known to have negative effects on fertility for both men and women. In women, smoking can lead to hormonal imbalances, damage to the reproductive organs, and a decrease in egg quality. For men, smoking can reduce sperm count, motility, and morphology. Quitting smoking is crucial for improving fertility outcomes. If you're struggling to quit, consider seeking support from healthcare professionals or support groups.

Alcohol and Fertility:

Excessive alcohol consumption can also have a detrimental effect on fertility. It can disrupt hormone levels in both men and women, leading to irregular menstrual cycles and decreased sperm quality. While moderate alcohol consumption is generally considered safe, it's best to limit alcohol intake when trying to conceive. The recommended limit is one drink per day for women and two drinks per day for men.

Poor Nutrition and Fertility:

A balanced and nutritious diet is essential for optimal fertility. Poor nutrition can lead to hormonal imbalances, irregular menstrual cycles, and decreased sperm quality. It's important to include a variety of fruits, vegetables, whole grains, lean proteins, and healthy fats in your diet. Additionally, maintaining a healthy weight is crucial for fertility. Consider consulting with a nutritionist or fertility specialist to develop a personalized diet plan.

By making positive lifestyle changes and addressing these unhealthy habits, you can significantly improve your chances of getting pregnant. Remember, small steps can make a big difference in your fertility journey. Prioritize your health and well-being to increase your chances of conceiving successfully.

Smoking and Fertility

Smoking and fertility are strongly linked, with smoking having detrimental effects on both male and female reproductive health. For couples trying to conceive, it is crucial to understand the negative impact that smoking can have on fertility and take steps to quit smoking for the sake of their reproductive success.

When it comes to female fertility, smoking can disrupt the delicate balance of hormones and interfere with the reproductive system. It can lead to irregular menstrual cycles, decrease egg quality, and increase the risk of miscarriage. Additionally, smoking can damage the fallopian tubes, making it difficult for the fertilized egg to travel to the uterus for implantation.

For men, smoking has been shown to reduce sperm count, motility, and overall sperm quality. The toxins in cigarettes can damage the DNA in sperm, leading to genetic abnormalities and an increased risk of infertility. Smoking can also impair erectile function and decrease libido, further impacting a couple's ability to conceive.

Quitting smoking is essential for couples trying to improve their chances of getting pregnant. Not only does it increase fertility, but it also improves overall health and reduces the risk of numerous other health problems. Here are some tips to help you quit smoking:

- Set a quit date and stick to it
- Find healthy alternatives to cope with cravings, such as chewing gum or snacking on fruits and vegetables
- Seek support from friends, family, or a support group
- Consider nicotine replacement therapy or prescription medications to help with withdrawal symptoms
- Avoid triggers and situations that tempt you to smoke
- Stay motivated by reminding yourself of the benefits of quitting, including improved fertility

Remember, quitting smoking is a journey, and it may take time and effort to overcome the addiction. However, the rewards of improved fertility and better overall health are well worth it. Seek support, stay committed, and take control of your reproductive future by saying goodbye to smoking.

Alcohol and Fertility

Understanding how alcohol consumption can affect fertility is crucial for couples who are trying to conceive. While enjoying a glass of wine or a cocktail occasionally may not significantly impact fertility, excessive alcohol consumption can have negative effects on both male and female fertility.

For women, alcohol can disrupt the hormonal balance necessary for regular ovulation and implantation of a fertilized egg. It can also increase the risk of miscarriage and decrease the chances of successful conception. In men, alcohol can lower sperm count, reduce sperm motility, and impair sperm quality, making it more difficult to achieve pregnancy.

It is important for couples trying to conceive to be aware of the recommended limits for alcohol consumption. The Centers for Disease Control and Prevention (CDC) advises women who are trying to get pregnant to abstain from alcohol completely. For men, it is recommended to limit alcohol consumption to no more than two drinks per day.

It is worth noting that alcohol can affect fertility even before conception occurs. Therefore, it is advisable for couples to adopt a healthy lifestyle and make positive changes well in advance of trying to conceive. By reducing or eliminating alcohol consumption, couples can improve their chances of successful conception and increase the likelihood of a healthy pregnancy.

Poor Nutrition and Fertility

Poor nutrition can have a significant impact on fertility. The food we eat plays a crucial role in the overall health of our bodies, including our reproductive systems. A healthy diet can help regulate hormones, improve egg quality, and support the development of a healthy embryo. On the other hand, a poor diet can lead to hormonal imbalances, inflammation, and oxidative stress, all of which can negatively affect fertility.

So, what should you eat to improve your chances of conceiving? Here are some tips for maintaining a healthy diet:

- Include plenty of fruits and vegetables in your meals. These are rich in antioxidants, which help protect your eggs and sperm from damage caused by free radicals.
- Choose whole grains over refined grains. Whole grains are a great source of fiber and essential nutrients that support reproductive health.
- Opt for lean proteins such as poultry, fish, and legumes. Protein is important for egg development and sperm production.
- Include healthy fats in your diet, such as those found in avocados, nuts, and olive oil. These fats help regulate hormone production and promote overall fertility.
- Avoid trans fats and limit your intake of saturated fats. These unhealthy fats can

increase inflammation and interfere with reproductive function.
- Stay hydrated by drinking plenty of water. Water is essential for maintaining optimal cervical mucus production, which is important for sperm survival and transportation.
- Limit your intake of processed foods, sugary snacks, and beverages. These can lead to weight gain, insulin resistance, and hormonal imbalances.

Remember, maintaining a healthy diet is not only important for fertility but also for the health of your future baby. By nourishing your body with the right nutrients, you are giving yourself the best chance of conceiving and having a healthy pregnancy.

Stress and Infertility

Stress and Infertility

When it comes to trying to conceive, stress can play a significant role in fertility. Research has shown that high levels of stress can interfere with the delicate hormonal balance needed for successful conception. The body's stress response, known as the "fight or flight" response, can disrupt the normal functioning of the reproductive system, making it more difficult to get pregnant.

But don't worry, there are techniques you can use to manage stress during the conception process. One effective method is to incorporate mind-body techniques into your daily routine. Meditation, yoga, and deep breathing exercises have been shown to reduce stress levels and improve fertility. These practices help to calm the mind, relax the body, and restore balance to the hormonal system.

Additionally, seeking counseling or joining a support group can be incredibly beneficial. Infertility can be emotionally challenging, and having a safe space to share your feelings and experiences can provide much-needed support and understanding. Talking to a professional therapist who specializes in fertility-related issues can also help you develop coping strategies and navigate the ups and downs of the journey.

Remember, managing stress is not only important for your fertility but also for your overall well-being. Taking care of yourself and finding healthy ways to cope with stress can make a significant difference in your fertility journey. So, take a deep breath, prioritize self-care, and know that you are not alone.

Mind-Body Techniques

Mind-Body Techniques

When it comes to reducing stress and improving fertility, mind-body techniques such as meditation and yoga can be incredibly beneficial. These practices not only help calm the mind and relax the body, but they also create a positive environment for conception.

Meditation, for instance, allows individuals to quiet their thoughts and focus on the present moment. By practicing meditation regularly, couples can reduce stress levels, promote emotional well-being, and enhance their overall fertility. It helps to create a sense of inner peace and balance, allowing the body to function optimally for conception.

Yoga, on the other hand, combines physical postures, breathing exercises, and meditation to promote relaxation and improve flexibility. It not only helps relieve tension and anxiety but also increases blood flow to the reproductive organs, supporting their healthy functioning. Additionally, certain yoga poses specifically target the pelvic area, stimulating the reproductive system and improving fertility.

Both meditation and yoga offer a holistic approach to reduce stress and improve fertility. They provide individuals with tools to manage their emotions, enhance their mind-body connection, and create a positive mindset during the conception process. By incorporating these mind-body techniques into their daily routine, couples can cultivate a sense of calmness, balance, and overall well-being, increasing their chances of successful conception.

Counseling and Support

Dealing with infertility can be an incredibly stressful and emotional experience for couples. The pressure to conceive can take a toll on their mental and emotional well-being. This is where counseling and support can play a crucial role in helping couples navigate the challenges of infertility.

Seeking professional help from a counselor or therapist who specializes in infertility can provide couples with a safe space to express their feelings, fears, and frustrations. A trained professional can offer guidance and support, helping couples develop healthy coping mechanisms and strategies to manage stress.

In addition to individual counseling, support groups can also be immensely beneficial for couples experiencing infertility-related stress. These groups provide a sense of community and understanding, as couples can connect with others who are going through similar struggles. Sharing experiences, discussing emotions, and receiving support from others who truly understand can help alleviate feelings of isolation and provide a sense of hope.

Support groups can be found both online and in-person, allowing couples to choose the format that best suits their needs. Online forums and social media groups provide a convenient platform for couples to connect with others from the comfort of their own homes. In-person support groups offer the opportunity for face-to-face interactions and personal connections.

It's important to remember that seeking counseling and joining support groups is not a sign of weakness, but rather an act of strength and self-care. Infertility can be a challenging journey, and having the right support system in place can make all the difference in maintaining emotional well-being and resilience.

Irregular Menstrual Cycles

Irregular menstrual cycles can significantly impact a woman's fertility and make it more challenging to conceive. Menstrual irregularities can include having periods that are too frequent, too infrequent, or unpredictable in terms of timing and duration. These irregularities can be caused by various factors, such as hormonal imbalances, polycystic ovary syndrome (PCOS), thyroid disorders, or underlying health conditions.

When periods are irregular, it becomes difficult to accurately predict ovulation, which is crucial for conception. Ovulation is the process in which a mature egg is released from the ovaries and is available for fertilization. If ovulation is irregular or absent altogether, it becomes challenging to time intercourse correctly to maximize the chances of pregnancy.

To regulate menstrual cycles and improve fertility, it is essential to address the underlying cause of the irregularities. This may involve lifestyle changes, medication, or other treatments. Here are some methods commonly used to regulate menstrual cycles:

- **Hormonal therapy:** In cases where hormonal imbalances are causing irregular periods, hormonal therapy may be prescribed. This can help regulate the menstrual cycle and promote regular ovulation.

- **Weight management:** Maintaining a healthy weight is crucial for hormonal balance and regular menstrual cycles. In cases where weight fluctuations or obesity contribute to irregular periods, adopting a balanced diet and engaging in regular exercise can help regulate the menstrual cycle.
- **Stress reduction:** Stress can disrupt hormonal balance and contribute to irregular periods. Engaging in stress-reducing activities such as yoga, meditation, or counseling can help regulate the menstrual cycle.
- **Herbal remedies:** Some herbal remedies, such as chasteberry or dong quai, are believed to have hormonal balancing properties and may help regulate menstrual cycles. However, it is essential to consult with a healthcare professional before using any herbal remedies.

It is important to remember that every woman's situation is unique, and what works for one person may not work for another. Consulting with a healthcare professional specializing in fertility can provide personalized guidance and treatment options to regulate menstrual cycles and improve the chances of conception.

Hormonal Imbalances

Hormonal Imbalances

Hormonal imbalances can significantly impact a woman's menstrual cycle and fertility. These imbalances occur when there is an abnormality in the production, regulation, or interaction of hormones in the body. Several factors can contribute to hormonal imbalances, including:

- Stress: Chronic stress can disrupt the delicate balance of hormones in the body, leading to irregular periods and difficulty conceiving.
- Polycystic Ovary Syndrome (PCOS): PCOS is a hormonal disorder characterized by the overproduction of androgens (male hormones) and the formation of cysts on the ovaries. This condition can disrupt ovulation and cause irregular menstrual cycles.
- Thyroid Disorders: An underactive or overactive thyroid gland can disrupt the production of hormones necessary for regular menstrual cycles.
- Obesity: Excess body weight can lead to hormonal imbalances, particularly an increase in estrogen levels, which can affect ovulation and menstruation.

Fortunately, there are potential treatments available to regulate the menstrual cycle and address hormonal imbalances. These treatments may include:

- Hormonal Birth Control: Oral contraceptives containing estrogen and progesterone can help regulate the menstrual cycle and balance hormone levels.
- Fertility Medications: Certain medications, such as Clomiphene citrate, can stimulate ovulation and regulate hormone production in women with hormonal imbalances.
- Lifestyle Modifications: Making healthy lifestyle changes, such as maintaining a balanced diet, exercising regularly, and managing stress levels, can help regulate hormone levels and improve fertility.
- Hormone Replacement Therapy: In some cases, hormone replacement therapy may be recommended to restore hormonal balance and regulate the menstrual cycle.

It is important for women experiencing hormonal imbalances to consult with a healthcare professional specializing in reproductive health. They can provide a comprehensive evaluation, diagnose the underlying cause of the imbalances, and recommend appropriate treatments tailored to individual needs.

Polycystic Ovary Syndrome (PCOS)

Polycystic Ovary Syndrome (PCOS)

Polycystic Ovary Syndrome (PCOS) is a common hormonal disorder that affects women of reproductive age. One of the main symptoms of PCOS is irregular periods, which can make it difficult for women to conceive. This condition is characterized by the presence of multiple small cysts on the ovaries, hormonal imbalances, and insulin resistance.

PCOS can disrupt the normal ovulation process, leading to irregular or absent periods. Without regular ovulation, it becomes challenging for women to get pregnant. However, there are strategies to manage PCOS and improve the chances of regular ovulation.

Diet and Lifestyle Modifications:

- Following a balanced and nutritious diet can help regulate hormone levels and improve fertility in women with PCOS. A diet rich in whole grains, lean proteins, fruits, and vegetables is recommended.
- Regular exercise can also play a crucial role in managing PCOS. Physical activity helps control insulin levels, promotes weight loss, and improves overall reproductive health.
- Managing stress is essential for women with PCOS. Stress can exacerbate hormonal imbalances and interfere with regular ovulation. Engaging in stress-reducing activities such as yoga, meditation, or counseling can be beneficial.

Medication:

In some cases, medication may be prescribed to manage PCOS and promote regular ovulation. Commonly prescribed medications include:

Medication	Purpose
Birth control pills	To regulate menstrual cycles and reduce androgen levels
Metformin	To improve insulin sensitivity and regulate hormone levels
Clomiphene citrate	To induce ovulation

Fertility Treatments:

If lifestyle modifications and medication alone are not effective, fertility treatments may be recommended for women with PCOS. These treatments aim to stimulate ovulation and increase the chances of pregnancy. Some common fertility treatments for PCOS include:

- Ovulation induction: This involves the use of medications such as clomiphene citrate or letrozole to stimulate ovulation.
- In vitro fertilization (IVF): IVF is a more advanced fertility treatment that involves fertilizing eggs with sperm in a laboratory and

then transferring the resulting embryos into the uterus.

- Other assisted reproductive technologies (ART): Depending on individual circumstances, other ART options such as intrauterine insemination (IUI) or intracytoplasmic sperm injection (ICSI) may be recommended.

It is important for women with PCOS to work closely with their healthcare providers to develop a personalized treatment plan. By managing PCOS effectively, women can improve their chances of regular ovulation and increase the likelihood of getting pregnant.

Low Sperm Count

Low sperm count, also known as oligospermia, is a common condition that can significantly impact a couple's chances of conception. It occurs when the semen contains fewer sperm cells than the normal range. There are several factors that can contribute to low sperm count, including:

- Hormonal imbalances
- Infections
- Varicocele (enlarged veins in the testicles)
- Genetic abnormalities
- Excessive heat exposure
- Smoking and alcohol consumption
- Poor diet and nutrition
- Stress and anxiety

Fortunately, there are techniques and lifestyle changes that can help improve sperm health and quantity. Here are some strategies to consider:

- **Healthy lifestyle habits:** Maintaining a healthy weight, exercising regularly, and avoiding excessive heat exposure (such as hot tubs or saunas) can help improve sperm count and quality.
- **Dietary changes:** Consuming a balanced diet rich in antioxidants, vitamins, and minerals can support sperm production. Foods like fruits, vegetables, whole grains, and lean proteins are beneficial for sperm health.
- **Supplements:** Certain supplements, such as zinc, selenium, and coenzyme Q10, may help improve sperm count and motility. However, it's important to consult with a healthcare professional before starting any new supplements.
- **Reducing exposure to toxins:** Avoiding exposure to harmful substances like pesticides, chemicals, and radiation can help protect sperm health.
- **Quitting smoking and limiting alcohol:** Smoking and excessive alcohol consumption have been linked to decreased sperm count and quality. Quitting smoking and

reducing alcohol intake can have a positive impact on fertility.
- **Stress management:** High levels of stress and anxiety can negatively affect sperm production. Engaging in stress-reducing activities like exercise, meditation, and yoga can help improve overall fertility.

If a couple is struggling with low sperm count and is unable to conceive naturally, they may consider seeking medical interventions such as assisted reproductive technologies (ART). These techniques, including in vitro fertilization (IVF) and intracytoplasmic sperm injection (ICSI), can help overcome low sperm count and increase the chances of successful conception.

It's important for couples experiencing low sperm count to consult with a fertility specialist who can provide personalized guidance and recommend the most appropriate treatments based on their specific situation.

Lifestyle Changes for Male Fertility

Lifestyle Changes for Male Fertility

When it comes to male fertility, making certain lifestyle modifications can greatly enhance sperm count and quality. By incorporating healthy habits into your daily routine, you can increase your chances of conception. Here are some key lifestyle changes to consider:

- **Diet:** A well-balanced diet rich in nutrients can promote optimal sperm production. Include foods that are high in antioxidants, such as fruits, vegetables, nuts, and seeds. These antioxidants help protect sperm from damage and improve their overall quality.
- **Exercise:** Regular physical activity can have a positive impact on male fertility. Engaging in moderate exercise, such as brisk walking or cycling, can help improve blood flow to the reproductive organs and enhance sperm production.
- **Avoid Heat Exposure:** High temperatures can negatively affect sperm production. Avoid hot baths, saunas, and tight-fitting underwear, as they can increase scrotal temperature and impair sperm health. Opt for loose-fitting, breathable clothing instead.

By implementing these lifestyle changes, you can optimize your fertility potential and increase the likelihood of successful conception. Remember, small adjustments can make a big difference when it comes to male fertility.

Medical Interventions for Male Infertility

When it comes to addressing low sperm count, there are several medical interventions available that can help improve male fertility. These interventions include medication and surgical procedures, which aim to enhance sperm production and quality.

One common medical treatment for male infertility is the use of medication. Certain medications, such as hormone therapies, can help regulate hormone levels and stimulate the production of sperm. These medications work by addressing hormonal imbalances that may be contributing to low sperm count. It is important to consult with a healthcare professional specializing in fertility to determine the most appropriate medication for individual circumstances.

In some cases, surgical interventions may be necessary to address low sperm count. Surgical procedures, such as varicocelectomy, can help correct anatomical abnormalities that may be obstructing sperm flow. This procedure involves the removal of enlarged veins in the scrotum, which can improve sperm production and quality. Another surgical option is testicular sperm extraction (TESE), which involves the extraction of sperm directly from the testicles for use in assisted reproductive techniques like in vitro fertilization (IVF).

It is important to note that the specific medical interventions for male infertility will vary depending on the underlying cause and individual circumstances. A thorough evaluation by a fertility specialist is crucial in determining the most appropriate treatment plan.

Blocked Fallopian Tubes

Blocked fallopian tubes can be a significant obstacle to achieving pregnancy. These tubes play a crucial role in the reproductive process, as they are responsible for carrying the egg from the ovary to the uterus. When the fallopian tubes are blocked, it prevents the egg from meeting the sperm, resulting in infertility.

There are several causes of blocked fallopian tubes. One common cause is pelvic inflammatory disease (PID), which is often caused by sexually transmitted infections such as chlamydia or gonorrhea. Other factors that can lead to blockages include endometriosis, previous pelvic surgeries, and adhesions or scar tissue from previous infections or surgeries.

To restore fertility in cases of blocked fallopian tubes, various treatments are available depending on the severity and location of the blockage. One common diagnostic procedure is hysterosalpingography (HSG), which involves injecting a dye into the uterus and fallopian tubes to detect any blockages. This procedure can help identify the location and severity of the blockage, allowing for more targeted treatment options.

If the blockage is minimal or located near the uterus, a minimally invasive surgical procedure called laparoscopy may be recommended. During this procedure, a small incision is made near the navel, and a tiny camera is inserted to visualize the fallopian tubes. The blockage can then be removed or repaired using specialized surgical tools.

In cases where the blockage is more severe or surgical intervention is not an option, in vitro fertilization (IVF) may be recommended. IVF bypasses the fallopian tubes altogether by fertilizing the egg with sperm in a laboratory setting and then transferring the resulting embryo into the uterus. This method can be highly effective for couples with blocked fallopian tubes.

It is important to consult with a fertility specialist to determine the best course of action for treating blocked fallopian tubes. They will be able to assess the specific circumstances and recommend the most suitable treatment option to restore fertility and increase the chances of conception.

Hysterosalpingography (HSG)

Hysterosalpingography (HSG) is a diagnostic procedure used to identify blocked fallopian tubes and potential treatments. It is a common test performed to evaluate the female reproductive system and determine the cause of infertility.

During an HSG, a contrast dye is injected into the uterus through the cervix. The dye then flows through the fallopian tubes, allowing the doctor to visualize the shape and structure of the tubes using X-ray imaging. If the dye does not flow freely through the tubes, it indicates a blockage.

HSG can help identify various causes of blocked fallopian tubes, such as scar tissue, adhesions, or structural abnormalities. Once the blockage is identified, appropriate treatment options can be considered.

The potential treatments for blocked fallopian tubes depend on the severity and location of the blockage. In some cases, minimally invasive procedures like laparoscopy can be performed to remove the blockage and restore fertility. In more complex cases, in vitro fertilization (IVF) may be recommended as an alternative method of achieving pregnancy.

It is important to discuss the results of the HSG with a fertility specialist who can provide personalized recommendations based on individual circumstances. HSG is just one of the many diagnostic tools available to help couples overcome infertility and achieve their dream of starting a family.

Surgical Interventions

Surgical Interventions

When it comes to addressing blocked fallopian tubes, surgical interventions can be a viable option for improving the chances of conception. One such surgical procedure is laparoscopy, which is a minimally invasive procedure that allows the surgeon to access the fallopian tubes and remove any blockages.

Laparoscopy involves making small incisions in the abdomen and inserting a thin, lighted instrument called a laparoscope. This allows the surgeon to visualize the fallopian tubes and identify any obstructions. Once the blockages are located, specialized surgical tools can be used to remove them, restoring the normal flow of eggs and sperm.

One of the advantages of laparoscopy is that it is less invasive than traditional open surgery, resulting in smaller incisions, reduced scarring, and a faster recovery time. It is typically performed under general anesthesia, and most patients can return home the same day.

It is important to note that laparoscopy may not be suitable for all cases of blocked fallopian tubes. The decision to undergo this procedure will depend on various factors, such as the severity and location of the blockages, as well as the overall health of the individual. Therefore, it is crucial to consult with a fertility specialist who can assess the specific situation and recommend the most appropriate course of action.

In some cases, laparoscopy may be combined with other surgical techniques, such as hysteroscopy, which allows for the examination and treatment of the uterine cavity. This comprehensive approach can further enhance the chances of conception by addressing any additional factors that may be contributing to infertility.

Overall, surgical interventions like laparoscopy offer hope for individuals with blocked fallopian tubes. By removing obstructions and restoring the normal function of the reproductive system, these procedures can significantly improve the likelihood of achieving a successful pregnancy. However, it is essential to seek professional medical advice

and guidance to determine the most suitable treatment
option based on individual circumstances.

Unexplained Infertility

Unexplained infertility can be a source of great frustration
for couples who are struggling to conceive. It is a diagnosis
given when all standard fertility tests come back normal, yet
pregnancy does not occur. This can leave couples feeling
confused and hopeless, wondering why they are unable to
conceive despite their best efforts.

One potential strategy for overcoming unexplained
infertility is to undergo comprehensive fertility testing to
identify any potential underlying causes that may have been
missed. This can include further investigation into hormone
levels, ovarian reserve, and sperm quality. By gaining a
deeper understanding of their fertility health, couples can
explore targeted treatment options that may increase their
chances of conception.

In addition to medical interventions, alternative therapies
can also be considered for unexplained infertility. Practices
such as acupuncture and herbal remedies have been used for
centuries to support reproductive health. While the scientific
evidence for these therapies may be limited, some couples
find them beneficial in reducing stress and promoting
overall well-being during the fertility journey.

Ultimately, the frustration of unexplained infertility can be
overwhelming, but it is important for couples to remember
that they are not alone. Seeking support from others who are

going through similar experiences can provide a sense of community and understanding. Support groups and therapy can offer a safe space for couples to express their emotions, gain valuable insights, and learn coping strategies to navigate the emotional challenges of infertility.

While the journey of unexplained infertility may be filled with uncertainty, it is essential for couples to prioritize self-care and stress management. Engaging in activities that bring joy and relaxation, such as exercise, meditation, or spending time in nature, can help alleviate the emotional burden. By taking care of their emotional well-being, couples can maintain a positive mindset and persevere in their quest for parenthood.

Fertility Testing and Diagnosis

When facing difficulties in conceiving, undergoing comprehensive fertility testing and diagnosis is crucial. These tests play a vital role in identifying potential underlying causes of infertility, enabling couples to explore appropriate treatment options. By understanding the importance of these tests, individuals can gain valuable insights into their reproductive health and make informed decisions about their fertility journey.

Fertility testing typically involves a series of evaluations for both partners. For women, this may include hormone level assessments, ovarian reserve testing, and imaging tests to examine the uterus and fallopian tubes. Men may undergo semen analysis to assess sperm count, motility, and morphology. Additionally, genetic testing may be recommended to identify any inherited conditions that could affect fertility.

Comprehensive fertility testing provides a comprehensive picture of the factors contributing to infertility. It helps determine if there are any hormonal imbalances, structural abnormalities, or genetic issues that need to be addressed. With this information, healthcare professionals can tailor treatment plans to address specific concerns and increase the chances of successful conception.

It is important to note that fertility testing can be a complex and emotionally challenging process. It is essential for couples to approach it with patience and support from healthcare providers. Understanding the significance of fertility testing and diagnosis empowers individuals to take control of their reproductive health and take necessary steps towards building their family.

Alternative Therapies

When facing the frustration of unexplained infertility, many couples turn to alternative therapies as a potential solution. These therapies, such as acupuncture and herbal remedies, offer a different approach to traditional medical treatments and may provide hope for those struggling to conceive.

Acupuncture:

Acupuncture is an ancient Chinese practice that involves the insertion of thin needles into specific points on the body. It is believed to help regulate the flow of energy, known as Qi, throughout the body. For couples dealing with unexplained infertility, acupuncture can potentially improve reproductive function by reducing stress, increasing blood flow to the reproductive organs, and balancing hormone levels.

Herbal Remedies:

Herbal remedies have been used for centuries in various cultures to address fertility issues. Certain herbs, such as chasteberry and maca root, are believed to have properties that can regulate hormonal imbalances and enhance reproductive health. However, it is important to consult with a qualified herbalist or healthcare professional before incorporating any herbal remedies into your fertility journey, as some herbs may interact with medications or have contraindications.

Other Alternative Therapies:

In addition to acupuncture and herbal remedies, there are other alternative therapies that couples may explore for unexplained infertility. These include:

- **Massage therapy:** Massage can help reduce stress and promote relaxation, which may have a positive impact on fertility.
- **Mind-body techniques:** Practices such as meditation, yoga, and deep breathing exercises can help manage stress and improve overall well-being.

- **Traditional Chinese medicine:** Traditional Chinese medicine encompasses various treatments, including acupuncture, herbal medicine, and dietary changes, to promote fertility.

It is important to note that alternative therapies should not replace medical advice or treatments. They can be used as complementary approaches to enhance overall fertility and well-being. Before starting any alternative therapy, it is recommended to consult with a healthcare professional who specializes in fertility to ensure it is safe and appropriate for your specific situation.

Assisted Reproductive Technologies (ART)

Assisted Reproductive Technologies (ART) have revolutionized the field of fertility treatment, offering hope to couples struggling to conceive. ART encompasses a range of advanced medical procedures that assist in achieving pregnancy when natural methods are not successful. One of the most well-known ART options is in vitro fertilization (IVF), which involves fertilizing an egg with sperm outside the body and then transferring the resulting embryo into the uterus.

IVF has proven to be highly effective in helping couples overcome infertility. The success rates of IVF vary depending on factors such as the age of the woman, the quality of the eggs and sperm, and the expertise of the fertility clinic. On average, the success rate for IVF is around 30% to 40% per cycle, with higher success rates for younger women and those using donor eggs.

In addition to IVF, there are other ART options available to couples. One such option is intracytoplasmic sperm injection (ICSI), which is often used in cases of male infertility. With ICSI, a single sperm is injected directly into the egg to facilitate fertilization. This technique has shown promising results, particularly for couples dealing with male factor infertility.

Another ART option is intrauterine insemination (IUI), also known as artificial insemination. In this procedure, prepared sperm is inserted directly into the woman's uterus during ovulation. IUI is often recommended for couples with unexplained infertility or mild male factor infertility.

It's important to note that the success rates of these ART options can vary depending on individual circumstances. Factors such as age, overall health, and the specific cause of infertility can all impact the chances of success. Consulting with a fertility specialist is crucial to determine the most suitable ART option for each couple.

IVF Process

The IVF process, or in vitro fertilization, is a complex and multi-step treatment option for couples struggling with infertility. It involves combining the egg and sperm outside of the body in a laboratory setting to facilitate fertilization.

Here is a breakdown of the steps involved in the IVF process:

1. **Ovarian Stimulation:** The first step in the IVF process is ovarian stimulation. This involves the administration of fertility medications to stimulate the ovaries to produce multiple eggs. Monitoring is done through blood tests and ultrasound to track the growth and development of the eggs.
2. **Egg Retrieval:** Once the eggs have reached the appropriate size, an egg retrieval procedure is performed. This is typically done under sedation or anesthesia. A thin needle is guided into the ovaries to collect the mature eggs.
3. **Sperm Collection:** On the same day as the egg retrieval, the male partner provides a semen sample. The sperm is then prepared in the laboratory to isolate the healthiest and most active sperm for fertilization.
4. **Fertilization:** The retrieved eggs and prepared sperm are combined in a laboratory dish for fertilization. The dish is then placed in an incubator to facilitate fertilization and embryo development.
5. **Embryo Culture:** The fertilized eggs, now embryos, are monitored and cultured in the laboratory for several days. This allows the

embryos to develop and grow before being transferred to the uterus.

6. **Embryo Transfer:** After the appropriate culture period, the embryos are transferred into the woman's uterus. This is typically done using a thin catheter that is guided through the cervix. The number of embryos transferred depends on various factors, including the woman's age and the quality of the embryos.

7. **Luteal Phase Support:** Following the embryo transfer, medications may be prescribed to support the luteal phase of the menstrual cycle. These medications help create an optimal environment for implantation and early embryo development.

8. **Pregnancy Test:** Approximately two weeks after the embryo transfer, a pregnancy test is done to determine if the IVF cycle was successful. This is typically a blood test that measures the levels of the pregnancy hormone, hCG.

It's important to note that not all IVF cycles result in pregnancy. The success rates of IVF can vary depending on factors such as the woman's age, the quality of the embryos, and the underlying cause of infertility. It's also common for couples to undergo multiple IVF cycles before achieving a successful pregnancy.

Overall, the IVF process can be a physically and emotionally demanding journey. It requires careful monitoring, coordination with healthcare professionals, and a strong support system. However, for many couples, IVF offers hope and the possibility of fulfilling their dream of starting a family.

Other ART Options

Other ART Options

When it comes to assisted reproductive technologies (ART), there are alternative methods that can be considered if in vitro fertilization (IVF) is not the right choice for you. These alternative options include intracytoplasmic sperm injection (ICSI) and intrauterine insemination (IUI).

Intracytoplasmic Sperm Injection (ICSI)

ICSI is a procedure that involves the direct injection of a single sperm into an egg. This technique is typically used when there are issues with sperm quality or quantity. By bypassing the need for the sperm to naturally penetrate the egg, ICSI increases the chances of fertilization. It is often recommended for couples with male factor infertility or those who have previously experienced failed fertilization attempts with IVF.

Intrauterine Insemination (IUI)

IUI is a less invasive ART option that involves placing washed and concentrated sperm directly into the uterus during the woman's fertile window. This procedure is commonly used for couples with unexplained infertility, mild male factor infertility, or cervical issues. It can also be used in combination with fertility medications to stimulate ovulation and increase the chances of conception. IUI is a simpler and more affordable option compared to IVF, making it a popular choice for many couples.

Comparing the Options

Factors	ICSI	IUI
Procedure Complexity	High	Low
Success Rates	Higher for severe male factor infertility	Lower compared to IVF, but higher than natural conception
Cost	Higher than IUI, but lower than IVF	Lower compared to IVF and ICSI
Indications	Male factor infertility, failed fertilization attempts with IVF	Unexplained infertility, mild male factor infertility, cervical issues

It is important to consult with a fertility specialist to determine which ART option is most suitable for your specific situation. Factors such as the cause of infertility, age, and overall health will be taken into consideration when determining the best course of treatment. With the advancements in reproductive medicine, there are various options available to help couples overcome infertility and fulfill their dream of starting a family.

Emotional and Psychological Impact

Emotional and Psychological Impact

Infertility can take a significant emotional toll on individuals and couples who are trying to conceive. The longing for a child and the disappointment of unsuccessful attempts can lead to feelings of sadness, frustration, and even guilt. It is important to acknowledge and address these emotions in order to maintain emotional well-being during the fertility journey.

One coping strategy is to seek support from others who are going through similar experiences. Support groups provide a safe space to share feelings, gain perspective, and receive encouragement. Talking to others who understand the challenges of infertility can help individuals and couples feel less alone and more supported.

Therapy is another valuable resource for addressing the emotional impact of infertility. A therapist can provide guidance and tools to navigate the complex emotions that arise during this time. They can help individuals and couples develop coping mechanisms and strategies for managing stress and anxiety.

Self-care is also crucial in maintaining emotional well-being. Engaging in activities that bring joy and relaxation can help reduce stress and improve overall mood. This can include hobbies, exercise, spending time in nature, or practicing mindfulness and meditation.

It is important for individuals and couples to remember that infertility does not define their worth or their ability to be parents. It is a challenging journey, but with the right support and coping strategies, it is possible to navigate the emotional and psychological impact of infertility and maintain hope for the future.

Support Groups and Therapy

Support groups and therapy can be invaluable resources for individuals and couples navigating the emotional challenges of infertility. Dealing with infertility can be an isolating and overwhelming experience, and connecting with others who are going through similar struggles can provide a much-needed sense of community and support.

Joining a support group allows individuals to share their experiences, fears, and frustrations in a safe and understanding environment. It provides an opportunity to connect with others who truly understand the emotional rollercoaster of infertility. Support groups can offer a space to vent, seek advice, and gain valuable insights from others who have faced similar obstacles.

Therapy, whether individual or couples counseling, can also be immensely beneficial for those dealing with infertility. A trained therapist can provide guidance and support in navigating the complex emotions that often accompany the fertility journey. Therapy can help individuals and couples develop coping mechanisms, manage stress, and improve communication.

In addition to emotional support, support groups and therapy can also provide practical resources and information. Members of support groups often share recommendations for fertility clinics, doctors, and alternative treatments. Therapists can offer guidance on different fertility treatment options and help individuals and couples make informed decisions about their reproductive health.

It's important to remember that seeking support and therapy is not a sign of weakness, but rather a proactive step towards emotional well-being during the infertility journey. Connecting with others who understand the unique challenges of infertility and having a professional guide can make a significant difference in coping with the ups and downs of trying to conceive.

Self-Care and Stress Management

Self-Care and Stress Management

During the fertility journey, it is crucial to prioritize self-care and implement effective stress management techniques to maintain emotional well-being. Dealing with infertility can be emotionally challenging, and taking care of oneself is essential to navigate this difficult time.

Here are some self-care practices and stress management techniques that can help individuals and couples cope with the emotional toll of infertility:

- **1. Prioritize self-care:** Make self-care a priority by engaging in activities that bring joy and relaxation. This can include hobbies, exercise, spending time with loved ones, or practicing mindfulness and meditation.
- **2. Seek support:** Joining support groups or seeking therapy can provide a safe space to share experiences, gain insights, and receive emotional support from others who understand the challenges of infertility.
- **3. Practice stress management techniques:** Implement stress management techniques such as deep breathing exercises, journaling, or engaging in activities that promote relaxation. These techniques can help reduce stress levels and promote emotional well-being.
- **4. Set boundaries:** It is important to set boundaries with others, especially when facing insensitive comments or questions about fertility. Communicate your needs and establish boundaries to protect your emotional well-being.

- **5. Take breaks:** Allow yourself to take breaks from fertility-related discussions and treatments. Engage in activities that provide a sense of normalcy and enjoyment, giving yourself time to recharge and rejuvenate.
- **6. Practice self-compassion:** Be kind to yourself and practice self-compassion. Remember that infertility is not your fault, and it is important to acknowledge and validate your emotions throughout the journey.

Remember, self-care and stress management are essential components of the fertility journey. By prioritizing self-care and implementing effective stress management techniques, individuals and couples can maintain emotional well-being as they navigate the challenges of infertility.

Frequently Asked Questions

- **Q: How does age affect fertility?**

  A: As women age, their fertility decreases due to a decline in the quality and quantity of eggs. Men also experience a decline in sperm quality as they get older. However, there are ways to improve chances of conception, such as seeking medical assistance or exploring assisted reproductive technologies.

- **Q: Can health conditions affect fertility?**

A: Yes, certain health conditions can interfere with fertility. Conditions like polycystic ovary syndrome (PCOS) and endometriosis can make it more difficult to conceive. However, there are potential treatments available to manage these conditions and increase the chances of successful conception.

- **Q: How does smoking affect fertility?**

A: Smoking can negatively impact fertility in both men and women. It can decrease sperm count and motility in men, and in women, it can affect the quality of eggs and increase the risk of miscarriage. Quitting smoking is highly recommended for couples trying to conceive.

- **Q: What is the connection between stress and infertility?**

A: High levels of stress can disrupt the hormonal balance in the body, affecting ovulation and sperm production. It is important to manage stress during the conception process through techniques such as meditation, yoga, and seeking counseling or support groups.

- **Q: How can irregular menstrual cycles impact fertility?**

A: Irregular periods can make it difficult to predict ovulation, which is essential for conception. Hormonal imbalances and conditions like PCOS can cause irregular periods. Regulating the menstrual cycle through hormonal treatments or lifestyle changes can improve fertility.

- **Q: What are some techniques to improve sperm health and quantity?**

  A: Lifestyle changes like maintaining a healthy diet, exercising regularly, and avoiding heat exposure (such as hot tubs or saunas) can enhance sperm count and quality. Medical interventions like medication or surgery may also be recommended depending on the underlying cause of low sperm count.

- **Q: What are the possible treatments for blocked fallopian tubes?**

  A: Diagnostic procedures like hysterosalpingography (HSG) can identify blocked fallopian tubes. Surgical interventions like laparoscopy can be performed to remove blockages and improve the chances of conception.

- **Q: What can be done for unexplained infertility?**

  A: Comprehensive fertility testing is important to identify any potential underlying causes. Alternative therapies like acupuncture or herbal remedies may also be explored. Seeking professional help and guidance is crucial in navigating the frustration of unexplained infertility.

- **Q: What are some common assisted reproductive technologies?**

  A: In vitro fertilization (IVF) is a widely used ART option. Other methods like intracytoplasmic sperm injection (ICSI) and intrauterine insemination (IUI) may also be recommended based on individual circumstances.

- **Q: How can individuals and couples cope with the emotional toll of infertility?**

  A: Joining support groups and seeking therapy can provide a valuable support system for individuals and couples experiencing infertility. Practicing self-care and stress management techniques is also important for maintaining emotional well-being throughout the fertility journey.

Have Questions / Comments?

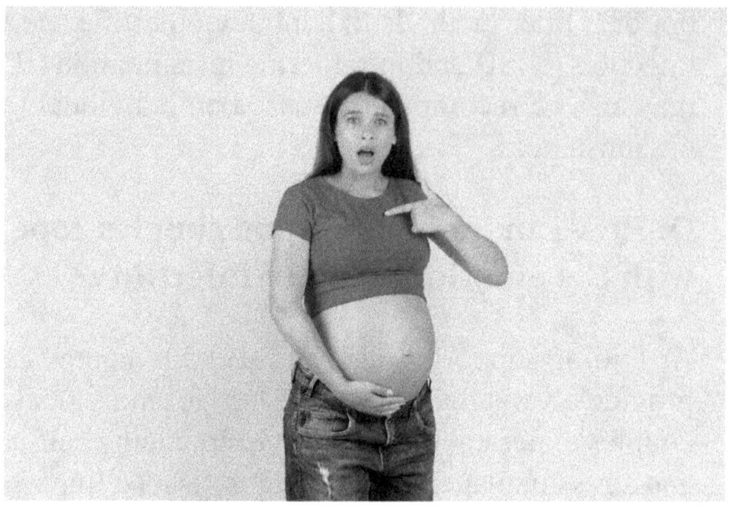

This book was designed to cover as much info as possible but I know I have probably missed something, or some new amazing discovery that has just come out.

If you notice something missing or have a question that I failed to answer, please get in touch and let me know. If I can, I will email you an answer and also update the book so others can also benefit from it.

Thanks For Being Awesome :)

Submit Your Questions / Comments At:

Get In Touch at Babydreamers.net

Get How To Be A Super Mom - 100% FREE

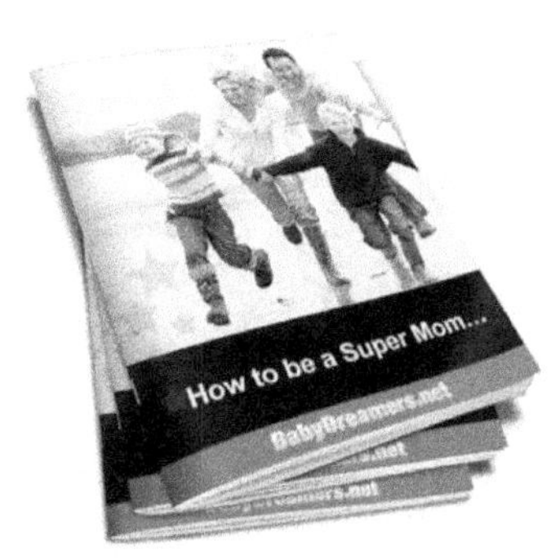

For being one of our amazing readers, we would love to offer you another book we have created, 100% free.

Being a mom is probably the most important job in the world – we've all heard that, and it's true. You're bringing up the next generation of wonderful, intelligent, loving, creative, responsible people.

We all want to be Super Mom and to be everything and do everything, but it this possible?

Being a Super Mom is possible, but you have to learn how to empower yourself to be the kind of Super Mom that you feel you need to be, keeping in mind that the title Super Mom doesn't mean the same thing to everyone.

Get How to be a Super Mom For Free at

BabyDreamers.net